Tighten Sagging Neck Skin

Look and Feel Younger and Sexier

Updated 2023 Edition!

Health and Anti-Aging Series

Angie Cruze

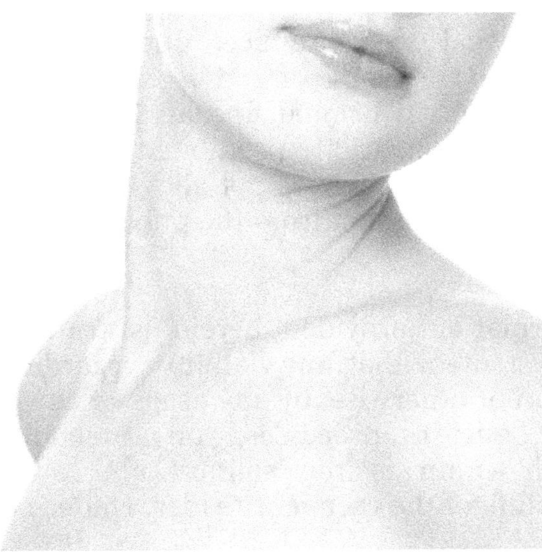

Contents

Introduction

Congratulations on downloading the book, **Tighten Sagging Neck Skin – Look and Feel Younger, Sexier.** Welcome to Angel Cruze's - *Health and Anti-Aging Series.*

This book explains what causes loose neck skin as you age. You'll learn the options available to look younger and more attractive. Surgery is a choice that can be expensive and may seem excessive to some people, but it can provide quick results. Other alternatives are creams (prices can vary from lower to relatively high), which tighten and revitalize your skin, or low-cost to no-cost strategies like improving nutrition and exercising. However, these can take longer to get results.

After reading this book, you will know why your neck skin has gotten loose and some options you have to combat its effects. Your increased knowledge will allow you to make an educated decision based on the risks you want to take, the effort and time you are willing to expend for improvement, and how much you want to spend.

Reading this book will help you make a better decision and prepare you for that visit to the doctor's office, cosmetic counter, grocery store, or gym.

So, get ready to throw away those turtle-necks!

Thanks again for downloading this book; I hope you enjoy it!

Why does your neck skin begin to sag and loosen as you age?

Did you know that the skin on your neck is thinner than your facial skin? Many people who spend a lot of money on beauty and skin care products often need to pay more attention to the skin on their necks. As a result, the skin on the neck often gives away their age, even though their faces look younger and fresh.

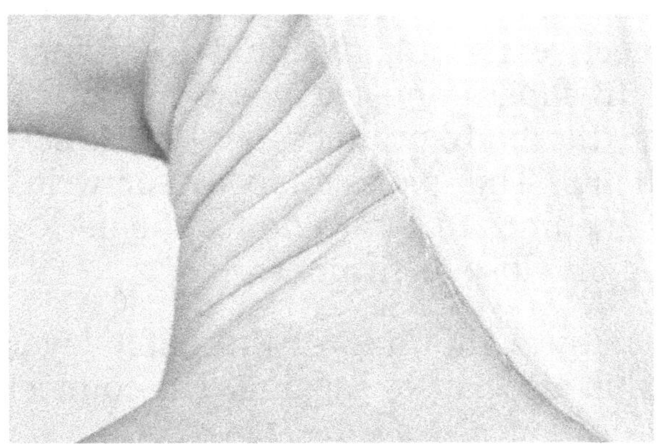

You do not need to look for unique skin care products for the neck because most items that help the face look younger can also be used on the neck. It is only natural for the skin to sag as you age, but there are cases when the occurrence happens earlier than usual. You can do something to slow down the aging process of your skin. First, you have to understand the causes of why the skin, specifically the neck skin, begins to sag and loosen as you age.

1. Your **genetic composition** significantly determines how your skin ages. You will likely follow the trend of how any of your parents' showed signs of aging. Everyone was born with natural levels of *elastin* (a protein that helps skin return to its original position when pinched) and *collagen* (the protein that is the main component of connective tissue), essential in giving the skin freshness and elasticity. As you grow older, the body produces less of these two elements. This paves the way for wrinkles and fine lines to show and for the neck skin to sag and lose its firmness.

The natural thinning of the outer layer of the skin also causes sagging. The connective tissue gets weaker as it happens, so the skin loses strength and elasticity.

2. **Stress** can take a significant toll on your skin. This can speed up the aging process, especially when you often expose yourself to factors that cause stress and anxiety. For one, your skin can develop rashes as it loses the strong barrier at its top layer, which prevents bacteria from entering the deeper layers of the skin. There is also a stress hormone called cortisol, which can shut down a part of your immune system. This makes you more prone to developing sicknesses like colds and flu. If you are often exposed to various stressors, your skin might develop problems, including warts, eczema, psoriasis, and shingles. In addition, negative thinking and being depressed will lead to deeper frown lines, which may be hard to counter and make you appear much older than your actual age.

Your skin will get dry when you are often stressed out. This is caused by the buildup of dead skin cells that make the skin look dull and dry. All these adverse effects of stress on your skin can speed up aging. If you don't do something about it early on, your skin will show signs of aging earlier.

3. **Too much sun exposure** can lead to premature skin aging. When the skin is often exposed to the sun's UV rays without sufficient protection, it gradually loses its elasticity, leading to saggy skin and wrinkles. For this reason, you must also avoid using a sun tanning bed to get an artificial tan because it exposes your skin to ultraviolet radiation. The artificial tanning device can help in medical procedures, such as treating psoriasis and dermatitis. However, when used for vanity, the effects will harm the skin in the long run.

4. **Smoking** can boost the aging process of your skin. This is because it narrows the blood vessels that distribute essential nutrients, oxygen, and vitamins to your skin. As a result, the skin loses its vibrancy, fine lines will appear, your neck skin will start to sag, and you will look older than your actual age. In addition, the bad habit of smoking depletes your system of Vitamin A, which is responsible for generating new skin cells and boosting collagen production.

Even if you don't smoke, too much exposure to secondhand smoke can lead to unhealthy skin.

4. **Losing weight** can also cause sagging of the skin. This is more evident when you lose much weight over a short period. Of course, the best way to counter this is to control your weight from the beginning by eating right and leading a healthy lifestyle; but if you're already overweight, use a slow, steady weight-loss program that includes exercise and nutrition.

Note: As you read through the following options, you may want to choose one or combine several. Always consult your doctor before taking action to improve your appearance or the look of your neck skin.

Option One – Surgical and Non-surgical Treatments

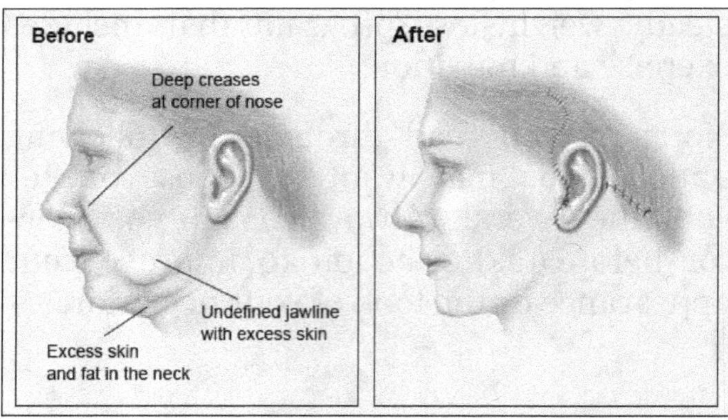

Surgery is an effective and fast way to enhance the appearance of your neck. It involves various procedures. Depending on your doctor's recommendation, you may need to undergo a process or a combination of multiple methods. It is best to consult with a good surgeon who can look into your problems and give you options on how to solve them. The usual neck skin problems include excess fat, turkey wattle neck, and too much skin.

The surgeon will look into your problem before they can provide a list of options. If the problem is a turkey wattle neck, the doctor may recommend surgery involving removing specific muscles. The surgery can also be done with the help of an endoscope or a small camera that will allow the surgeon to make minor cuts to eliminate the problem. When the neck looks full, the doctor may recommend a non-surgical option, like Botox, to relax the situation's cause without needing a knife. You will be given a choice regarding the anesthesia used during the surgery. This will depend on whether you want to remain conscious during the procedure.

Here is an overview of the standard non-surgical and surgical procedures that can help bring back your neck skin's beauty.

1. **Ultrasound Therapy.** "Utherapy" is a non-surgical treatment that uses micro-focused ultrasound to generate a thermal effect under the skin.

You may wonder what the diff-erence is between Utherapy and Laser skin therapy.

Both can be used for skin tightening, but Laser focuses energy on the skin's surface, while Ultherapy targets deep below the skin (3 mm and 4.5 mm beneath the surface), lifting and tightening from the inside out.

This effect helps your body create new **collagen** by bypassing the skin's surface through focused ultrasound energy at the right amount, depth, and temperature. The results appear over 2 to 3 months and last a year or more until the natural aging process again begins to reduce collagen production. You may visit *ultherapy.com* for more information on Ultherapy.

2. **Liposuction.** Your doctor may recommend that you undergo surgical procedures. If liposuction is the only procedure you will go through, the operation might take up to an hour. The procedure is common and preferred by many people because it is not only effective but it is also less expensive.

This procedure can be done in two ways - Tumescent and Ultrasonic Assisted or UAL. In both these procedures, the surgery will begin through the tiny incisions beneath the chin or behind the earlobes.

When undergoing Tumescent procedure, a localized pain medicine will be injected into your system, along with epinephrine. Then, when your fat is already swollen, a cannula, a device like a tube, will be inserted. The process of breaking up and vacuuming the fat will then begin.

A special cannula (tube) is used in the UAL procedure. Before suctioning the fat, it liquefies it through the energy it sends out, which comes in sound waves.

After the doctor completes the procedure, Tumescent or UAL, the incisions will be closed through tape. You will be required to wear a compression garment for several days. It is only normal to suffer from swelling and develop bruises during recovery. You must allot a week to heal and return to your usual routine. After this time frame, you will also notice the improvements the procedure has made on your neck skin. This can cost $3,000 or more if other problems are discovered during the process. This is cosmetic surgery. This means that your insurance probably won't shoulder the expenses.

The neck skin will be contoured and smooth when the healing is complete. Unfortunately, there are cases when swelling continues even after the wound has healed. You can only undergo this procedure if you are healthy because it can be risky if you have other serious health issues.

2. **Trimming.** This is typically done to those who have too much neck skin. After giving you anesthesia, the excess skin will be trimmed and lifted into place. This might last from two to four hours. The cuts will be secured with stitches or tissue glue when the doctor is done. You will be given a compression bandage that you have to wear for at least one week or up until the wounds he healed.

3. **Platysmaplasty surgery.** This is highly recommended to those with a turkey wattle or loose neck muscles. For your doctor to reach the platysma or neck muscle, incisions will be made beneath the

chin or behind the ears. The problematic muscles will then be manipulated accordingly or removed if required. The doctor may opt for permanent sutures to hold the tissue in place.

4. **Neck lift and facelift.** Combining these procedures can solve excess skin problems on the neck, chin, and jowls. You will be given anesthesia before an incision is made behind the ear. This will make the muscles tighter after getting rid of the excess skin. Both procedures are done to eliminate the signs of aging in the face and neck.

A modified procedure for combining these processes is recommended for those with excessive skin problems. The modified version eliminates the fatty deposits, removes the excess skin, and positions the tissues more youthfully.

Before you undergo any of these procedures, you must follow your doctor's advice on preparing for it.

First, you must avoid taking certain medications that might contribute to excessive bleeding during the operation.

Tell your doctor if you have any allergic reactions to anesthesia and other drugs so that they can give you a safer option.

If you are a smoker, you must stop a month before the surgery and during the healing process after the operation.

Give yourself sufficient time to heal. Refrain from forcing yourself to go back to work immediately after undergoing the operation. Healing might take a week or even longer, depending on what procedures were done and how your body coped with it. During this period, make sure that you eat healthy food. You should also wear loose, comfortable clothes with limited contact with your wound.

Ensure you have easy access to ice packs, towels, and thermometers useful when you suffer from side effects such as bleeding, swelling, and fever. You must also have an antibacterial ointment handy to help eliminate itching without scratching the affected part.

When there is an infection, you must first check if you have a fever. Your doctor has to be informed if you have a fever and if you notice any unusual discharge from your wound.

The other side effects of the surgery include bruising, burning or tingling sensations, numbness, and tightness.

The cost of the procedures varies depending on who the surgeon is, the medications, and the operations that you were required to undergo. The usual neck lift procedures may cost from $3,000 to $8,000. You can talk to your doctor about a suitable financing option to make paying for the cost you might incur easier.

Option Two – Creams

The problems with aging neck skin may also be improved through anti-aging and other beauty creams. While most facial creams can also be applied to the neck, certain products are specifically formulated to address the problems of your neck skin.

Neck tightening creams contain three key components including:

- **Peptides** – Proteins that help the production of collagen (the main component of connective tissue).

- **Plant Stem Cells** – Cells that repair and strengthen the skin's barrier from environmental stresses through anti-oxidant and anti-inflammatory prop-erties.

- **Antioxidants** – Nutrients that protect and revitalize the skin from endogenous and exogenous oxidative stresses by scavenging free radicals. They may benefit the skin by preventing or slowing aging and cell damage.

Creams may include ingredients such as:

- **Retinol** is a vitamin A derivative that can increase collagen production and thicken the skin.

- **DMAE, or dimethylaminoethanol**, is a natural chemical antioxidant in fatty fish. It is said to improve skin tone and texture and plump and firm the skin, causing the muscles to contract.

- **Vitamin B3,** formulated as niacinamide, has been proven to improve skin elasticity.

- **Vitamin C,** formulated into

L-ascorbic acid tightens skin by increasing collagen production and helps prevent certain enzymes from degrading some types of collagen.

- **Vitamin E,** or alpha-tocopherol, is used smooth the skin and help it retain moisture.

Disclaimer: Consult your doctor and use skin creams at your own risk.

You would be surprised at the number of creams available. For example, an internet search for "neck tightening creams" yielded 1,620,000 results. Yes, that's 1 million, six hundred thousand.

According to **Consumer Review** *https:// consumereview.org*, here are three of the top neck creams:

1. **Agelyss Neck Firming Cream.** Rated Excellent. It contains the highest percentage of active ingredients (10%), 5 top quality patented and trademarked ingredients, and doesn't contain parabens, hormones,

or artificial fragrances. Price: About $69 for a 1 oz bottle.

2. **Neocutis® Neo Firm Neck & Décolleté Tightening Cream.** Rated Good. It contains Glycolic Acid, a proprietary Peptide Blend, and additional Vitamin-C for intensive skin nourishment, moisturizing, and tightening. A 1.69 oz bottle will run you about $135.

3. **Replenix® Lifting + Firming Neck Cream.** Rated OK. It contains Biomimetic Ceramides, Peptides, Niacinamide, and Edelweiss flower extract. Paraben-free and gluten-free, this neck cream considers the sensitivities of many skin types. A 1.7 oz bottle will run you about $77.

Finding a neck skin tightening cream that works for you can be frustrating and expensive if you only use trial and error and don't get lucky quickly. Instead, ask for recommendations from your doctor, or listen to friends and family who have tried the products. Read reviews and spend time researching. By doing some homework, you'll save time and money.

Out of the hundreds of neck-firming creams available, here are a few others for you to consider:

Lacura Firming Face and Neck Cream. This may be the least expensive of the neck creams that many people have proven safe and effective. This can be bought for less than $10. This works with all skin types, but the results can only be visible after several months of continued use.

L'Oreal Advanced Revitalift Face & Neck Day Cream. The product is reasonably priced at $10-15 per jar. It gives your skin 24 hours of moisture as it works in the renewal cells, reduce fine lines, and makes the skin tighter and firmer. In addition, this product contains Retinol, a type of Vitamin A that boosts the growth of new skin cells; pro-lastyl, which makes the skin more elastic and firmer; and Criste Marine Extract, which encourages skin renewal and smoothes wrinkles.

Aside from being easy on the budget, the product has a milder smell than many other products. Visible results will be evident after a few months. During the first few days of use, your skin will feel softer and smoother. This is non-greasy and can be worn under makeup. This is safe and effective, but some people develop rashes after trying it. Try it out in a small area of your arm before using the product. This way, you will be sure you are not allergic to any of its components.

Bare Minerals Extra Firming Neck Cream. In 2023, depending on where you purchase it, this cream is available for $50 to $100 for a 3.4-ounce jar. This all-in-one cream provides care to delicate neck skin by locking in moisture, lifting the skin, and restoring its youthful look. Many of those who have tried this said that the cream is absorbed quickly by the skin and does not leave any residue. As a result, the effects take longer to be seen, making the skin firmer.

StriVectin Tightening Neck Cream. This is available for around $95 for a jar of 1.7 ounces. Some people say that this works fast, and the results can be seen after a short period. The product has undergone clinical testing to prove its effectiveness in making the neck skin firm and smooth.

Dermagist. This is among the most expensive brands of neck creams. A 60 ml bottle of Dermagist costs around $65. Its topical formula can be applied to the neck every day. Many people who have tried using the product testified that they felt the instant firmness of their neck skin after only several applications. Even after you have stopped using the product, it continues to work by reducing the formation of wrinkles.

The Dermagist Neck Restoration Cream combines effective ingredients to solve neck skin problems. It has Matrixyl, which works by smoothening deep wrinkles, the Stem Cells that help in regenerating damaged skin cells, Hyaluronic Acid that locks in moisture in the skin, Sesaflash that makes the skin firmer, and Shea Butter that also helps in making the skin firmer and hydrated.

Clarins Extra-Firming Neck Cream. This is highly rated by many people who have tried using the product but is considered expensive at about $96 for a 2.5 oz tube. Reviews have said it effectively makes the skin firmer and less saggy. It is hydrating and does not leave skin with a greasy feel. This can be applied once daily; the results will be seen after several days. This can also produce long-term results through continued use. Its only setback is its strong fragrance, but the product is safe and effective.

Option Three – Nutrition

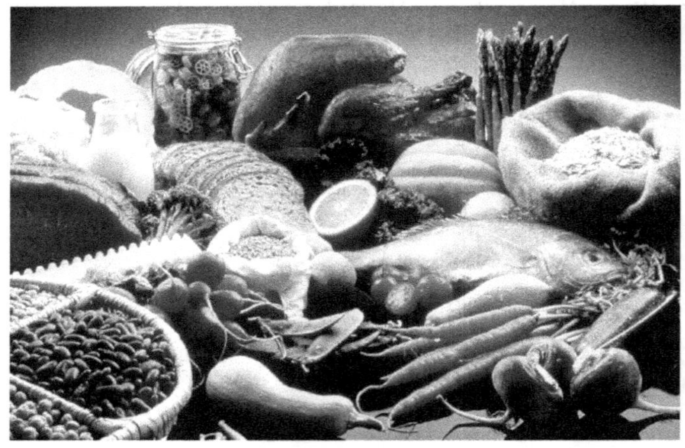

Skin problems and imminent signs of skin aging can also be brought on by the food you eat. So, if you want a low-cost option to address your neck skin concerns, try changing your diet to improve your skin tone and firmness.

Therefore, the best skin solution is eating a balanced diet. For healthier skin, remember these crucial pointers related to your food intake.

What foods should you avoid?

First, reduce your intake of SUGAR and carbohydrates! Sugars like glucose and fructose lead to glycation, a natural bodily process that causes sugar molecules to adhere to your skin's collagen and elastin proteins. These proteins being weighed down by sugar molecules results in inflammation and signs of skin aging. In addition, the process of glycation causes advanced glycation end-products (AGEs) to form, making collagen rigid and losing its ability to keep skin firm. Also, the inflamemation caused by AGEs dries the skin.

High-sugar foods like soda, white bread, cupcakes, candy, and table sugar should be reduced or avoided.

Second, reduce your intake of fatty foods. They also cause glycation and AGE formation. They include french fries, fish sticks, fried chicken, chicken tenders, onion rings, and other foods fried in vegetable oil.

What foods are good for skin and general health?

You must supply your system with a good dose of **Vitamin A**. This is more important if you have other health conditions like thyroid disease and diabetes. Vitamin A can be acquired from dairy products. For example, low-fat yogurt has a high Vitamin A content and live bacteria that benefit your intestines. With healthy digestion, you are also assured of healthy-looking skin.

Provide your system with food **rich in antioxidants, such** as plums, strawberries, and blueberries. These fruits also contain phytochemicals that help in protecting the cells from damage. As a result, you can guard yourself against early forms of skin aging. The other food items that contain high antioxidants include beans, prunes, artichokes, and pecans.

There are food items that help in keeping the cell membranes healthy, which is essential for the skin to be able to hold and retain moisture. These items include foods rich in **essential fatty acids**, such as flax D, walnuts, canola oil, and salmon.

You must supply your system with sufficient **selenium levels** to effectively counter the effects of sun exposure. This can be done by including food items, such as muffins, cereals, whole wheat bread, tuna, and turkey, into your diet.

Instead of coffee, it is healthier to **drink green tea**. It contains anti-inflammatory properties that can help in reducing the adverse effects of exposure to UV rays. This can reduce the risk of developing skin cancer. Aside from being taken orally, some products use this as an active ingredient, which can be applied directly to the skin.

You must make it a habit of drinking plenty of water daily. It keeps your body hydrated and your skin naturally moisturized. In addition, water helps your system eliminate toxins and absorb the nutrients you get from food.

Your body needs a good dose of **Vitamin B Complex,** which is essential for keeping your skin and hair healthy. This can be obtained from food items such as eggs, oats, rice, and bananas.

Will protein in your diet help in making your skin healthier? Protein is essential for your body to replace dead cells and to repair damaged cells and tissue. The amount of protein your body needs depends on weight and physical activity. The higher the level of your physical activities, the more protein you will need to help repair and rebuild your muscles.

Foods that may be used for *good* protein intake include salmon, eggs, plain Greek yogurt, almonds, tofu, lentils, goji berries, walnuts, and hemp seeds.

Avoid frying or deep-fried cooking if you eat red meat or poultry. Also, avoid foods with additives, hormones, and antibiotics.

Option Four – Exercise

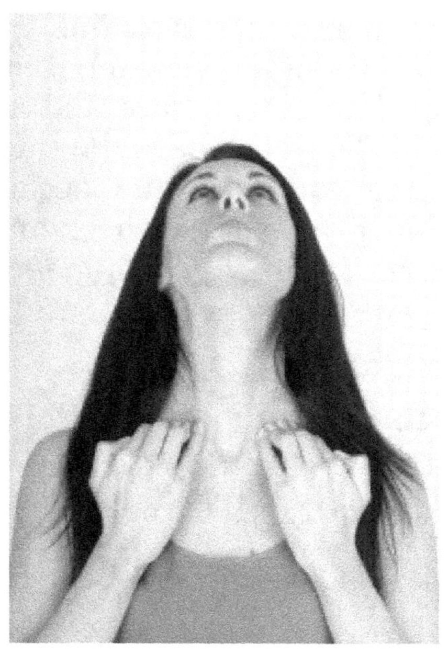

Aside from following a healthy diet, it is essential that you exercise regularly. These techniques can make your body fitter and your skin healthier and firmer. The best thing about combining diet and exercise is that this is low-cost and effective. For example, exercising and eating right will improve the appearance of your loose neck skin but will benefit your entire body without buying expensive beauty products or undergoing cosmetic procedures.

You'll find many videos online regarding face and neck **yoga**. The exercises help to release tension in your face and neck and reduce pain. They also have the side benefit of tightening your face and neck skin by strengthening the face and neck muscles. A link to Face Yoga is _www.goodhousekeeping.com/health/wellness/g26828923/face-yoga-exercises/_.

What other kinds of exercises can tighten loose neck skin? You can do the following exercises regularly. These exercises can help address your problem with loose neck skin and alleviate neck pain.

1. **Dorsal Glide.** This can be done easily while you lay on your back. While in this position, you must put a small towel or an ice pack beneath your neck. You can also do this while sitting or standing if you keep your head straight. Your goal is to stretch

the back of your neck. You must tuck your chin as you perform the gliding process of your head towards your back. Do not force yourself to glide farther when you already feel the pain from the motion.

When you reach the point where your head and neck muscles are still comfortable, hold the position. Count to six. Slowly return to your original position, relax for a few seconds, and repeat the process up to twelve times.

2. **Hands-on head.** This is a form of an isometric exercise. It uses force to resist an object until the tension builds up without making any movements. This exercise aims to make the muscles of your neck stronger. You must begin by keeping your neck straight and your vision straight ahead.

Start the exercise on the right side of the neck. You put your right hand on the right side of your head. Press your head with your hand while the hand resists the pressure. During the process, your neck muscles will tighten. Press your hand firmly and ensure your head cannot move to either side. Hold the position for six counts, relax for several seconds, and then repeat.

You use the same steps but use your left hand to exercise the other side of your neck this time.

To exercise your upper back, intertwine your fingers and place your hands on the back of your head. Next, press your head into your hands, making sure that your head does not tip at the back. Hold this position for six counts, relax, and repeat the process.

For the muscles at the front of the neck, you place the heels of your two hands against your forehead. Press your head firmly against your hands, ensuring your head does not tip forward. Hold this position for six counts, relax for a few seconds, and then repeat.

3. **Neck stretch.** First, you must relax your shoulders. It will help if you hold onto something for support, like a chair or your thighs. Keep your shoulder down while you try to lean away from your body. You then tilt your head toward your shoulder. Hold this in place for 15 seconds, then relax before repeating the process.

Conclusion

Thank you again for downloading this book!

Our goal was to improve your knowledge of why your neck skin has gotten loose (the aging process and natural reduction in elastin and collagen production, genetic composition, stress, sun exposure, smoking, and rapid weight loss) and some of your options to combat its effects (surgical and non-surgical treatments including ultrasound therapy, liposuction, trimming, platysmaplasty, neck and face lift). You also learned about skin treatments using creams, including their ingredients and how they work. Finally, you learned of some less invasive natural therapies, such as improving your nutritional intake or exercises that focus on improving the appearance of your neck skin.

It's time to take what you've learned and act on it. Tighten that loose neck skin and become the healthier, more attractive, and more confident person you deserve to be.

Use what you've learned:

1. Stop smoking.
2. Reduce sun exposure.
3. Improve your diet and nutrition.
4. Lose weight slowly in conjunction with everything else on this list.
5. Exercise regularly.
6. If it's right for you, consider creams and surgical and non-surgical solutions.

I truly hope this book helps you take positive action to improve your neck's appearance and make you look and feel younger. However, consult your doctor before deciding what action to take.

Now it's up to you...

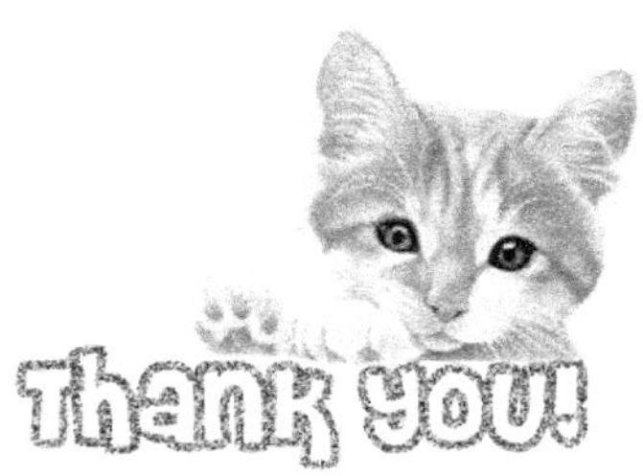

Finally, if you enjoyed this book, I'd like to ask you for a favor. Would you be kind enough to *leave a review for this book on Amazon*? It'd be greatly appreciated!

Thank you, and good luck!

These are the other books currently in our **Health and Anti-Aging series**. Check them out on Amazon.

Facial Skin Guide to a Softer, Clearer and Firmer Face

A Guide to Varicose Vein Prevention and Treatment

A Guide to Looking Younger by Tightening Up Loose, Sagging Arm Skin

- **How to Get Back the Slim, Toned Arms of Your Youth**

A Guide to Understanding and Preventing Heart Disease

Kidney Stones - Prevention and Treatment

If you have any suggestions on a future topic or would like to get on our email list for future updates, please email <u>manilaz@outlook.com</u>. Please make your email subject contains "Health and Anti-Aging."

Much, much more to come in the series.

Check out another book on Amazon by this publisher:

Mortgage Refinancing: 5 Mortgage Loan Secrets You Need to Know Before Talking with a Lender